DIABETES COOKBOOK FOR EVERYONE

The Complete Diet Cookbook Guide to Manage Types 2 Diabetes and Reverse Prediabetes

Fortune Flourish

Copyright Page

Copyright © 2024 by Fortune Flourish

TABLE OF CONTENTS

INTRODUCTION

Welcome to "Eating Well with Diabetes: A Nutritious Journey to Better Health." This cookbook is not just a collection of recipes; it's a guide, a companion, and a source of inspiration for anyone navigating the complexities of managing diabetes through diet. Diabetes is a serious condition that affects millions of people worldwide.

Whether you've recently been diagnosed or have been living with diabetes for years, one thing remains constant; the importance of nutrition in managing your health. What you eat plays a crucial role in controlling blood sugar levels, reducing the risk of complications, and promoting overall well-being.

At the heart of this cookbook is the belief that eating well with diabetes doesn't mean sacrificing flavor or enjoyment. Instead, it's about making informed choices, embracing variety, and finding balance in your meals. From hearty breakfasts to satisfying dinners, from savory snacks to decadent desserts, each recipe in this book has been carefully crafted to meet the needs of individuals with diabetes while tantalizing the taste buds.

Before we delve into the delicious recipes that await you, let's take a moment to understand the relationship between diabetes and nutrition. Diabetes is a condition characterized by high blood sugar levels, either due to insufficient insulin production (Type 1 diabetes) or the body's inability to use insulin effectively (Type 2 diabetes).

While genetics and other factors play a role in its development, lifestyle choices, particularly diet, can significantly impact the course of the disease. Carbohydrates, in particular, have a direct effect on blood sugar levels. However, not all carbohydrates are created equal.

The concept of glycemic index (GI) and glycemic load (GL) helps us understand how different foods affect blood sugar levels. Foods with a low GI and GL are digested and absorbed more slowly, leading to gradual rises in blood sugar levels and better glucose control.

In this cookbook, you'll find a wealth of recipes featuring low-GI ingredients, helping you keep your blood sugar stable throughout the day.

But managing diabetes isn't just about carbohydrates. Protein and fat also play important roles in regulating blood sugar levels and promoting satiety. By including a balance of these macronutrients in your meals, you can optimize your diet for diabetes management while enjoying a diverse array of flavors and textures.

Meal planning is another key component of diabetes management. By carefully selecting ingredients and portion sizes, you can create meals that not only taste great but also support your health goals. In this cookbook, you'll find practical tips and strategies for meal planning, along with sample meal plans to guide you on your journey. Above all, "Eating Well with Diabetes" is about empowerment.

It's about taking control of your health and making choices that nourish your body and soul. Whether you're cooking for yourself, your family, or friends, these recipes are designed to inspire creativity in the kitchen and bring joy to the table. So, turn the page, pick up your apron, and let's embark on this nutritious journey together. With each recipe you try, may you discover the pleasure of eating well with diabetes and the power of nourishing your body with love and care.

CHAPTER ONE

"Understanding Diabetes and Nutrition"

Diabetes is a complex and challenging condition that requires careful management, and one of the most important aspects of this management is nutrition. What you eat can have a significant impact on your blood sugar levels, overall health, and quality of life. In this section, we'll explore the relationship between diabetes and nutrition, providing you with the knowledge and tools you need to make informed dietary choices.

What is Diabetes?

Diabetes is a chronic metabolic disorder characterized by high blood sugar levels, either due to insufficient insulin production, ineffective use of insulin, or both. Insulin, a hormone produced by the pancreas, plays a crucial role in regulating blood sugar levels by facilitating the uptake of glucose from the bloodstream into cells, where it can be used for energy.

There are several types of diabetes, with the most common being Type 1 diabetes, Type 2 diabetes, and gestational diabetes.

Type 1 diabetes: This an autoimmune condition in which the immune system mistakenly attacks and destroys the insulin-producing cells in the pancreas.

Type 2 diabetes: This typically develops later in life and is characterized by insulin resistance, where the body's cells become less responsive to insulin.

Gestational diabetes: Occurs during pregnancy, although it normally goes away after childbirth, it might raise the chance of Type 2 diabetes in the future.

The Role of Nutrition in Diabetes Management

Nutrition plays a crucial role in diabetes management for several reasons. First and foremost, what you eat directly impacts your blood sugar levels. Carbohydrates, in particular, have the most significant effect on blood sugar, as they are broken down into glucose during digestion.

Monitoring carbohydrate intake and choosing carbohydrates that have a minimal impact on blood sugar, such as whole grains, fruits, vegetables, and legumes, can help regulate blood sugar levels and prevent spikes and crashes. In addition to carbohydrates, protein and fat also play important roles in diabetes management.

Protein and fat have less of an immediate effect on blood sugar compared to carbohydrates but can still influence blood sugar levels, especially when consumed in large quantities. Including lean sources of protein, such as poultry, fish, tofu, and legumes, and healthy fats, such as avocados, nuts, seeds, and olive oil, can help stabilize blood sugar levels and promote satiety

The Importance of a Healthy Diet for Diabetes Management"

Managing diabetes is a multifaceted endeavor that involves various lifestyle modifications, with diet playing a central role. A healthy diet is not just beneficial but crucial for effectively managing diabetes and mitigating its associated risks. In this section, we'll delve into the significance of adopting a nutritious diet tailored to the needs of individuals with diabetes.

Blood Sugar Control

One of the primary goals of diabetes management is to regulate blood sugar levels within a healthy range. Diet plays a pivotal role in achieving this objective. During digestion, carbohydrates in particular are converted into glucose, which directly affects blood sugar levels. Choosing the right carbohydrates—those with a low glycemic index (GI) and glycemic load (GL)—can help prevent sudden spikes and dips in blood sugar levels.

Incorporating whole grains, fruits, vegetables, and legumes into the diet provides a steady source of energy while minimizing blood sugar fluctuations.

Weight Management

Maintaining a healthy weight is essential for individuals with diabetes, as excess body weight can exacerbate insulin resistance and increase the risk of complications. A balanced diet that emphasizes nutrient-dense foods, such as lean proteins, whole grains, fruits, and vegetables, can support weight management efforts. By focusing on portion control, consuming fewer calories than expended, and making nutritious food choices, individuals with diabetes can achieve and maintain a healthy weight, thereby improving overall health outcomes.

Heart Health

Heart disease is a common complication of diabetes and a leading cause of mortality among individuals with the condition. Adopting a heart-healthy diet can help mitigate the risk of cardiovascular complications associated with diabetes.

A diet rich in fruits, vegetables, whole grains, lean proteins, and healthy fats, such as those found in fish, nuts, seeds, and olive oil, can help lower cholesterol levels, reduce inflammation, and promote heart health. Limiting the intake of saturated and trans fats, sodium, and added sugars is also important for protecting cardiovascular health.

Prevention of Complications

Diabetes increases the risk of developing various complications, including neuropathy, nephropathy, retinopathy, and foot ulcers. A well-balanced diet, coupled with regular physical activity and medication adherence, can help prevent or delay the onset of these complications. Consuming foods rich in vitamins, minerals, and antioxidants, such as fruits, vegetables, whole grains, and lean proteins, supports overall health and reduces the risk of diabetes-related complications.

Quality of Life

Beyond its physiological benefits, adopting a healthy diet can significantly enhance the quality of life for individuals with diabetes. By fueling the body with nutritious foods that provide sustained energy and supporting overall well-being, a healthy diet can improve mood, increase energy levels, and promote a sense of vitality.

Additionally, maintaining a healthy diet fosters a positive relationship with food, empowering individuals to make informed choices that prioritize their health and longevity.

In conclusion, a healthy diet is a cornerstone of diabetes management, offering numerous benefits for blood sugar control, weight management, heart health, prevention of complications, and overall quality of life. By embracing a diet rich in nutrient-dense foods and mindful eating habits, individuals with diabetes can optimize their health outcomes and thrive in their journey towards wellness.

How This Cookbook Can Help?

A diabetes diet cookbook can be incredibly helpful for managing diabetes because it provides recipes and meal plans tailored to controlling blood sugar levels. Here's how it can help:

Balanced Meals: A good cookbook will offer a variety of recipes that are balanced in terms of carbohydrates, protein, and fats. This balance is crucial for keeping blood sugar levels stable.

Portion Control: Many people with diabetes struggle with portion control, which can affect blood sugar levels. A cookbook will often provide portion sizes and nutritional information, helping you manage your intake more effectively.

Healthy Ingredients: A diabetes diet cookbook will focus on using healthy, whole ingredients that are low in added sugars and unhealthy fats. This can help improve overall health and reduce the risk of complications associated with diabetes.

Controlled Carbohydrates: Carbohydrate management is key for people with diabetes, as carbohydrates directly affect blood sugar levels. A cookbook designed for diabetes will often include recipes with controlled carbohydrate content to help you manage your intake.

Meal Planning: Planning meals in advance is important for managing diabetes. A cookbook can provide meal plans and ideas for breakfast, lunch, dinner, and snacks, making it easier to stick to a healthy eating routine.

Variety and Flavor: Eating the same foods over and over again can get boring. A diabetes cookbook offers a wide variety of recipes and flavors to keep your meals interesting and enjoyable, making it easier to stick to your dietary goals.

Expert Guidance: Many diabetes cookbooks are written by experts in the field of nutrition and diabetes management. They often include valuable information about managing diabetes through diet, as well as tips and tricks for success.

Overall, a diabetes diet cookbook can be an invaluable resource for anyone looking to better manage their diabetes through healthy eating. It provides practical guidance, delicious recipes, and helpful tips to support your journey to better health.

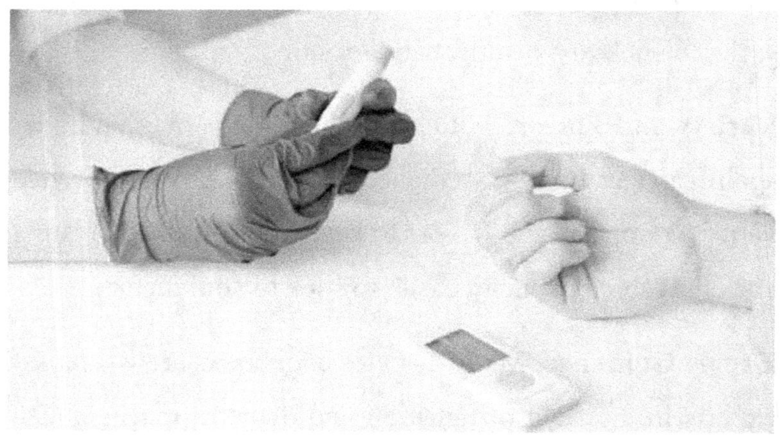

CHAPTER TWO

Basics of Diabetes Nutrition

The basics of diabetes nutrition revolve around managing blood sugar levels through mindful eating and making healthy food choices. Here are some fundamental principles:

Balanced Meals: Aim for well-balanced meals, with a mix of healthy fats, proteins, and carbs. This balance helps to regulate blood sugar levels and provides sustained energy throughout the day.

Carbohydrate Management: Carbohydrates have the most direct impact on blood sugar levels, so it's important to monitor your carbohydrate intake. Focus on complex carbohydrates like whole grains, fruits, vegetables, and legumes, which are digested more slowly and cause a gradual rise in blood sugar.

Healthy Fats: Incorporate healthy fats, such as those found in nuts, seeds, avocados, and olive oil, into your diet. These fats can help improve insulin sensitivity and keep you feeling full and satisfied.

Lean Protein: Include lean sources of protein, such as poultry, fish, tofu, and legumes, in your meals. Protein helps to stabilize blood sugar levels and keeps you feeling full between meals.

Fiber-Rich Foods: Choose fiber-rich foods like fruits, vegetables, whole grains, and legumes, as they can help slow down the absorption of sugar into the bloodstream and improve blood sugar control.

Limit Added Sugars and Refined Carbs: Minimize your intake of added sugars, sugary beverages, and refined carbohydrates like white bread, white rice, and sugary snacks. These foods can cause rapid spikes and dips in blood sugar levels.

Regular Meal Timing: Try to eat meals and snacks at regular intervals throughout the day to help regulate blood sugar levels and prevent extreme fluctuations.

Stay Hydrated: To maintain general health and keep hydrated, sip lots of water throughout the day. Avoid sugary drinks and opt for water, herbal tea, or other low-calorie beverages.

Portion control is important to prevent blood sugar increases caused by overindulging, so be mindful of portion sizes. Use measuring cups, food scales, or visual cues to help you control portion sizes, especially for carbohydrate-rich foods.

Monitor and Adjust: Monitor your blood sugar levels regularly and adjust your diet as needed based on your readings. Work closely with your healthcare team, including a registered dietitian, to develop a personalized nutrition plan that meets your individual needs and goals.

By following these basic principles of diabetes nutrition, you can better manage your blood sugar levels, improve your overall health, and reduce the risk of diabetes-related complications.

Carbohydrates, Proteins and Fats:

What you need to know

Understanding carbohydrates, proteins, and fats is essential for maintaining a healthy diet and overall well-being. This is what you need to know about each macronutrient:

Carbohydrates:

Carbohydrates are the body's primary source of energy and are found in a variety of foods, including fruits, vegetables, grains, legumes, and dairy products.

Carbs are classified into two primary categories: simple carbs, or sugars, and complex carbohydrates, or starches and fiber.

Simple carbohydrates are quickly digested and can cause rapid spikes in blood sugar levels. They are found in foods like candy, soda, and processed snacks.

Complex Carbs: The release of energy from complex carbs is more gradual and lasts longer. Foods such as fruits, vegetables, legumes, and whole grains contain them.

It's important to choose carbohydrates that are high in fiber and nutrients and to monitor portion sizes to help regulate blood sugar levels, especially for individuals with diabetes.

Proteins:

Building and mending tissues, producing hormones and enzymes, and bolstering immune system function all depend on proteins.

Protein is found in foods like meat, poultry, fish, eggs, dairy products, tofu, tempeh, legumes, nuts, and seeds.

Proteins are made up of amino acids, some of which are considered essential because the body cannot produce them and they must be obtained from the diet.

It's important to consume a variety of protein sources to ensure you get all the essential amino acids your body needs.

Fats:

Fats are another important source of energy and are essential for the absorption of fat-soluble vitamins (A, D, E, and K), hormone production, and providing insulation and protection for organs.

There are different types of fats, including saturated fats, unsaturated fats (monounsaturated and polyunsaturated), and trans fats.

Saturated fats are found in animal products like meat and dairy, as well as some plant-based oils like coconut oil and palm oil. They should be consumed in moderation as they can raise cholesterol levels.

Unsaturated fats: These are found in foods like nuts, seeds, avocados, olive oil, and fatty fish. They are considered heart-healthy fats and should be included as part of a balanced diet.

Trans fats: These are artificial fats found in processed foods like fried foods, baked goods, and margarine. They should be avoided as they can increase the risk of heart disease.

It's important to choose healthy fats and limit the intake of saturated and trans fats to support heart health and overall well-being.

Balancing carbohydrates, proteins, and fats in your diet can help you maintain energy levels, support muscle growth and repair, regulate blood sugar levels, and promote overall health and vitality. It's important to focus on whole, nutrient-dense foods and to consume them in appropriate portions to meet your individual nutritional needs.

Glycemic Index and Glycemic Load Explained

The glycemic index (GI) and glycemic load (GL) are two measures used to assess the impact of carbohydrate-containing foods on blood sugar levels. Here's an explanation of each:

Glycemic Index (GI):

The glycemic index is a scale that ranks carbohydrate-containing foods based on how much they raise blood sugar levels compared to a reference food, usually pure glucose or white bread, which is assigned a value of 100.

Foods with a high GI (70 or above) cause blood sugar levels to rise quickly, leading to a rapid increase in insulin production. Examples include white bread, white rice, sugary cereals, and most processed snack foods.

Foods with a low GI (55 or below) cause a slower, more gradual rise in blood sugar levels and are typically digested and absorbed more slowly. Examples include most fruits and vegetables, whole grains, legumes, and nuts.

Foods with a moderate GI (56-69) fall somewhere in between and have a moderate impact on blood sugar levels.

Glycemic Load (GL):

While the glycemic index ranks individual foods, the glycemic load takes into account both the quality and quantity of carbohydrates in a serving of food.

To determine a food's glycemic load, multiply its glycemic index by the total number of carbs in a serving, then divide the result by 100.

Foods with a high glycemic load (20 or above) may still cause a significant increase in blood sugar levels, even if they have a relatively low glycemic index because they contain a large amount of carbohydrates per serving. Examples include watermelon and white potatoes.

Foods with a low glycemic load (10 or below) have a smaller impact on blood sugar levels per serving, even if they have a high glycemic index because they contain fewer carbohydrates per serving. Examples include lentils and most non-starchy vegetables.

In conclusion, the glycemic load considers both the quantity and quality of carbohydrates in a portion of food, whereas the glycemic index assesses how rapidly a diet containing carbs elevates blood sugar levels. Both measures can be useful for managing blood sugar levels and choosing foods that promote stable energy levels and overall health.

Portion Control and Meal Planning Tips.

Portion control and meal planning are crucial aspects of managing diabetes, and a diabetes cookbook can provide helpful guidance in these areas. Here are some tips for portion control and meal planning using a diabetes cookbook:

Use Measuring Tools: Invest in measuring cups, spoons, and a food scale to accurately measure portion sizes. This will help you control your carbohydrate intake and prevent overeating.

Follow Serving Sizes: Pay attention to serving sizes listed in the recipes of your diabetes cookbook. Stick to these recommended portions to help manage your blood sugar levels.

Plate technique: For portion control, use the plate technique as a reference. Distribute the non-starchy veggies on half of your plate, lean protein on one quarter, and carbs on the other quarter. This balanced approach can help regulate blood sugar levels and promote overall health.

Pre-portion Snacks: Prepare snacks in advance and portion them into individual servings. This makes it easier to grab a healthy snack on the go without overindulging.

Meal Prep: Spend some time each week meal prepping to ensure you have healthy, portion-controlled meals ready to go. Use your diabetes cookbook to plan meals for the week and batch cook items like grains, proteins, and vegetables.

Include Fiber: Choose recipes from your diabetes cookbook that are high in fiber, such as those containing whole grains, legumes, fruits, and vegetables. Fiber helps regulate blood sugar levels and promotes satiety, reducing the likelihood of overeating.

Plan for Variety: Aim for variety in your meals by choosing recipes from your diabetes cookbook that incorporate different types of proteins, carbohydrates, and vegetables. This not only keeps meals interesting but also ensures you're getting a wide range of nutrients.

Keep Track of Carbs: If you're managing your carbohydrate intake, use your diabetes cookbook to iden.,tify recipes with appropriate carbohydrate counts. Keep track of your carbohydrate intake throughout the day to help maintain stable blood sugar levels.

Consider Leftovers: Many recipes from your diabetes cookbook can be doubled or tripled to provide leftovers for future meals. By doing this, you can guarantee that you always have healthy alternatives available and save time.

Listen to Your Body: Pay attention to hunger and fullness cues, and stop eating when you're satisfied. Eating mindfully and in moderation can help prevent overeating and promote better blood sugar control.

By implementing these portion control and meal planning tips with the help of your diabetes cookbook, you can better manage your blood sugar levels and support overall health and well-being.

Reading Food Labels for Diabetes-Friendly Choice

Reading food labels is essential for making diabetes-friendly choices and managing blood sugar levels effectively. Here's a guide to reading food labels for individuals with diabetes:

Serving Size: Start by looking at the serving size listed at the top of the food label. All the information on the label, including the number of calories and nutrients, is based on this serving size. Be mindful of portion sizes to avoid overeating.

Total Carbohydrates: Pay close attention to the total carbohydrates listed on the food label. Carbohydrates have the most significant impact on blood sugar levels, so it's crucial to monitor your intake. Look for foods with lower carbohydrate content, especially if you're counting carbs to manage your diabetes.

Fiber: Check the fiber content of the food. Fiber is beneficial for individuals with diabetes because it can help regulate blood sugar levels and improve overall health. Choose foods that are high in fiber and low in added sugars and refined carbohydrates.

Sugars: Look at the amount of sugars listed on the food label. Be aware that this includes both natural sugars (like those found in fruit or dairy) and added sugars (like high fructose corn syrup or cane sugar). Try to limit foods that are high in added sugars, as they can cause spikes in blood sugar levels.

Ingredients List: Review the ingredients list to see what the food is made of. Ingredients are listed in descending order by weight, so the first few ingredients make up the majority of the product. Avoid foods with added sugars, refined grains, and unhealthy fats. Look for whole, minimally processed ingredients.

Saturated and Trans Fat: Check the amount of saturated and trans fats in the food. These fats can increase the risk of heart disease, which is already elevated in individuals with diabetes. Choose foods that are low in saturated and trans fats and higher in healthy fats like monounsaturated and polyunsaturated fats.

Sodium: Keep an eye on the sodium content of packaged foods. High sodium intake can contribute to high blood pressure and other health issues, so it's essential to limit your intake. Choose foods that are lower in sodium or opt for low-sodium varieties whenever possible.

Nutrient Claims: Be cautious of nutrient claims on food packaging, such as "sugar-free" or "low-fat." These claims can sometimes be misleading, so it's important to read the entire food label and consider the overall nutritional value of the product.

Use Percent Daily Value (%DV): The %DV tells you how much of a specific nutrient one serving of the food provides in relation to the daily recommended intake. Use the %DV to help you understand the nutritional content of the food and make informed choices.

By carefully reading food labels and making diabetes-friendly choices, you can better manage your blood sugar levels and support overall health and well-being.

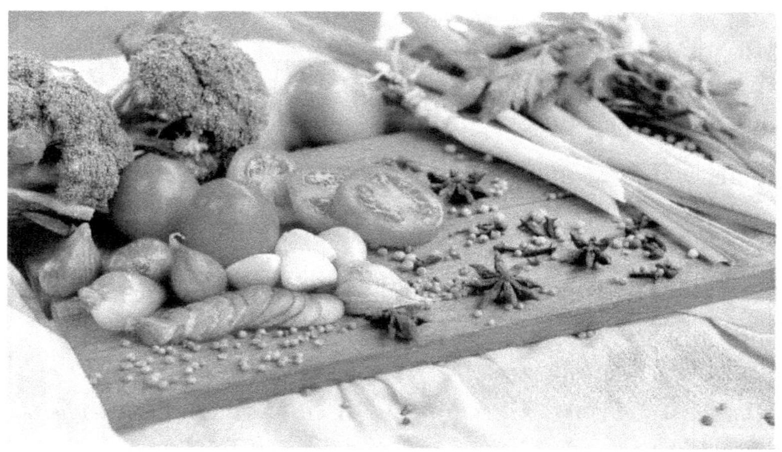

CHAPTER THREE

Breakfast Recipes

1. Low-Glycemic Breakfast Ideas:

1,1 Greek Yogurt Parfait: Layer Greek yogurt with mixed berries and a sprinkle of nuts or seeds for added crunch. Greek yogurt is low in carbohydrates and high in protein, making it a great option for managing blood sugar levels.

1.2 Vegetable Omelette: Whip up an omelette with your choice of vegetables, such as spinach, bell peppers, onions, and tomatoes. Pair it with a slice of whole grain toast for a satisfying, low-glycemic breakfast.

1.3 Chia Seed Pudding: Mix chia seeds with unsweetened almond milk and a touch of vanilla extract. Let it sit in the refrigerator overnight to thicken, then top with sliced strawberries and a sprinkle of cinnamon in the morning. Chia seeds are high in fiber and low in carbohydrates, making this a nutritious and filling breakfast option.

2. High-Fiber Breakfast Options:

2.1 Overnight Oats: Combine rolled oats with unsweetened almond milk, chia seeds, and your favorite fruits (such as bananas or berries) in a jar. Let it sit in the refrigerator overnight, and enjoy a creamy, high-fiber breakfast in the morning.

2.2 Whole Grain Pancakes: Make pancakes using whole grain flour and add mashed bananas or grated apples to the batter for natural sweetness and extra fiber. Top with a dollop of Greek yogurt and a drizzle of honey or maple syrup.

2.3 Quinoa Breakfast Bowl: Cook quinoa in unsweetened almond milk and top with sliced almonds, diced apples, and a sprinkle of cinnamon. Quinoa is a complete protein and high in fiber, making it an excellent choice for a nutritious breakfast.

3. Quick and Easy Breakfasts for Busy Mornings:

3.1 Smoothie: Blend together frozen berries, spinach, Greek yogurt, and a scoop of protein powder for a quick and nutritious breakfast on the go. Add a splash of unsweetened almond milk to achieve your desired consistency.

3.2 Whole Grain Toast with Nut Butter: Spread almond or peanut butter on whole grain toast and top with sliced bananas or berries for a simple and satisfying breakfast option.

3.3 Egg Muffins: Preheat the oven to 350°F (175°C) and whisk together eggs, diced vegetables, and a sprinkle of cheese. Pour the mixture into muffin tins and bake for 20-25 minutes until set. These egg muffins can be made ahead of time and reheated for a quick and protein-packed breakfast.

These breakfast recipes offer a variety of options for different dietary needs and preferences, including low-glycemic, high-fiber, and quick and easy options for busy mornings. Enjoy experimenting with these recipes and adapting them to suit your taste preferences and nutritional goals.

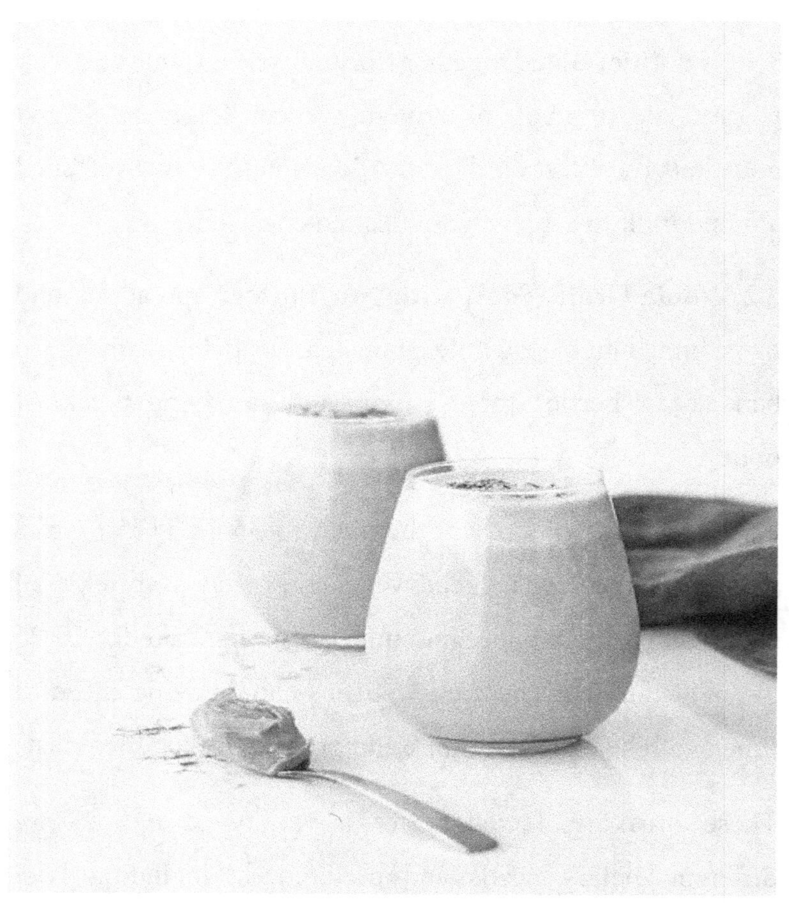

CHAPTER FOUR

Lunch Recipes

1. Salads and Wrap

1.1. Grilled Salmon Salad

A bed of mixed greens, cherry tomatoes, cucumber slices, and avocado is topped with a grilled salmon fillet. Use a simple vinaigrette composed of lemon juice and olive oil to dress.

1.2 Quinoa and Black Bean Bowl:

Cooked quinoa mixed with black beans, diced bell peppers, corn, and cilantro. Top with grilled chicken or tofu for added protein and drizzle with a lime-cumin dressing.

1.3 Turkey and Hummus Wrap:

Whole grain wrap filled with sliced turkey breast, hummus, shredded carrots, cucumber, and baby spinach leaves. Serve with a side of sugar snap peas or sliced bell peppers.

.1.4 Mediterranean Chickpea Salad:

Chickpeas tossed with diced cucumbers, cherry tomatoes, red onion, Kalamata olives, and feta cheese. Garlic, oregano, lemon juice, and olive oil are used to dress.

1.5 Grilled Chicken Caesar Wrap:

Grilled chicken breast slices wrapped in a whole grain tortilla with romaine lettuce, cherry tomatoes, grated Parmesan cheese, and Caesar dressing made with Greek yogurt.

1.6 Tuna and White Bean Salad:

Canned tuna mixed with white beans, diced red onion, cherry tomatoes, and chopped parsley. Toss with a basic vinaigrette consisting of Dijon mustard, red wine vinegar, and olive oil.

1.7 Asian-Inspired Chicken Salad:

Shredded rotisserie chicken tossed with shredded cabbage, carrots, bell peppers, and edamame. Drizzle with a ginger-soy dressing and top with sliced almonds or sesame seeds.

1.8 Egg and Avocado Breakfast Burrito (also great for lunch!):

Scrambled eggs wrapped in a whole grain tortilla with mashed avocado, diced tomatoes, spinach leaves, and a sprinkle of feta cheese.

1.9 Vegetable Stir-Fry with Tofu:

Stir-fried tofu with a variety of colorful vegetables such as bell peppers, broccoli, snap peas, and carrots. Season with garlic, ginger, and low-sodium soy sauce, and serve over brown rice or quinoa

These lunch ideas offer a balance of carbohydrates, protein, and healthy fats to help keep blood sugar levels stable and provide sustained energy throughout the day. Feel free to alter them to suit your dietary requirements and tastes.

2. Soups and Stews for Satisfying Meals to manage blood sugar

2.1 Vegetable Lentil Soup:

A hearty soup made with lentils, carrots, celery, onions, tomatoes, and spinach. Seasoned with herbs like thyme and bay leaves for flavor. Lentils provide a good source of protein and fiber, which can help stabilize blood sugar levels.

2.2 Chicken and Vegetable Quinoa Soup:

A nutritious soup featuring cooked quinoa, diced chicken breast, carrots, celery, bell peppers, and kale. Add garlic, ginger, and a splash of low-sodium soy sauce to taste. Quinoa adds fiber and protein to the soup, helping to keep you full and satisfied.

2.3 Black Bean and Vegetable Chili:

A flavorful chili made with black beans, diced tomatoes, bell peppers, onions, and zucchini. Seasoned with chili powder, cumin, and smoked paprika for a rich, smoky flavor. Black beans are a great source of fiber and protein, which can help regulate blood sugar levels.

2.4 Turkey and White Bean Soup:

A comforting soup made with ground turkey, white beans, diced tomatoes, carrots, celery, and onions. Seasoned with herbs like rosemary and thyme. Turkey provides lean protein while white beans add fiber, making this soup a balanced meal for managing blood sugar.

2.5 Vegetable and Chickpea Curry:

A warming curry stew made with chickpeas, cauliflower, bell peppers, onions, and spinach in a flavorful coconut milk-based broth. Seasoned with curry powder, turmeric, and ginger for added depth of flavor. Chickpeas are rich in fiber and protein, which can help stabilize blood sugar levels.

2.6 Italian Wedding Soup:

A classic Italian soup featuring meatballs made from lean ground turkey or chicken, acini di pepe pasta, spinach, carrots, and celery in a savory chicken broth. Packed with protein, vegetables, and whole grains, this soup is a satisfying option for managing blood sugar.

2.7 Tomato Basil Soup with Lentils:

A comforting tomato soup made with lentils, diced tomatoes, onions, carrots, and celery. Seasoned with fresh basil, garlic, and a splash of balsamic vinegar for brightness. Lentils add protein and fiber to this delicious soup.

2.8 Mushroom Barley Soup:

A hearty soup made with pearl barley, sliced mushrooms, carrots, onions, and celery in a savory vegetable broth. Seasoned with thyme and bay leaves for aromatic flavor. Barley is whole grain rich in fiber, which can help stabilize blood sugar levels.

These soups and stews are packed with nutritious ingredients like vegetables, lean protein, and whole grains, making them excellent choices for managing blood sugar levels while still enjoying delicious and satisfying meals.

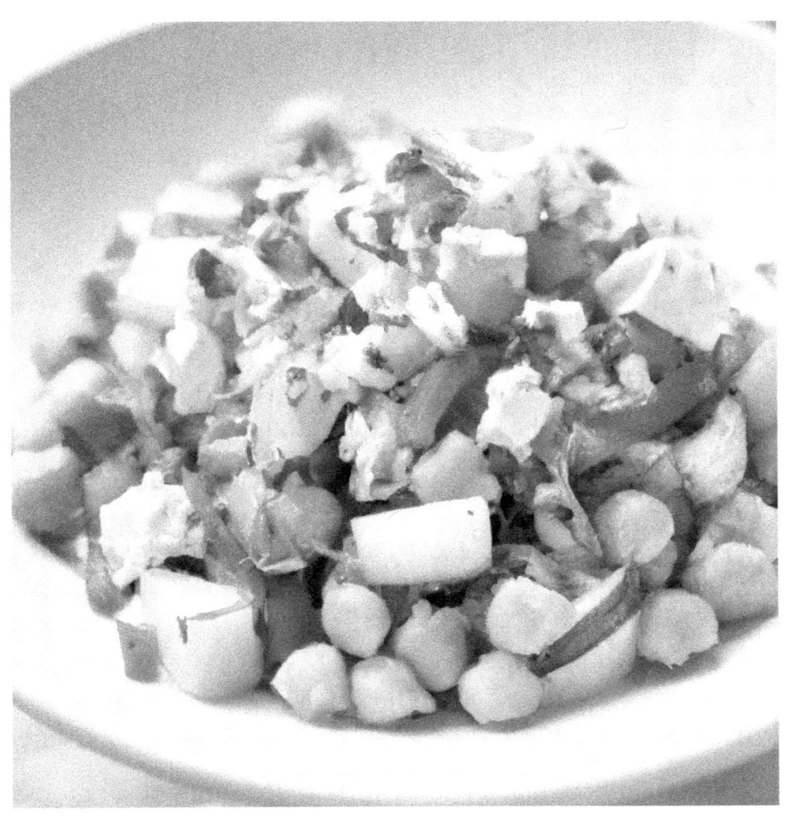

Mediterranean chickpea salad

CHAPTER FIVE

Dinner recipes

1. Flavorful and Nutritious Dinners:

1.1 Grilled Lemon Herb Salmon:

Marinate salmon fillets in a mixture of lemon juice, olive oil, minced garlic, and fresh herbs like dill and parsley. Grill until cooked through and serve with roasted asparagus and quinoa pilaf.

1.2 Stuffed Bell Peppers:

Halve bell peppers and remove seeds, then fill with a mixture of cooked quinoa, black beans, corn, diced tomatoes, onions, and spices. Top with shredded cheese and bake until peppers are tender and filling is heated through.

1.3 Chicken and Vegetable Stir-Fry:

Stir-fry sliced chicken breast with a variety of colorful vegetables such as bell peppers, broccoli, carrots, and snap peas in a ginger-garlic sauce. Serve over brown rice or cauliflower rice for a nutritious and satisfying meal.

1.4 Baked Eggplant Parmesan:

Bread slices of eggplant in a mixture of breadcrumbs and Parmesan cheese, then bake until golden and crispy. Layer with marinara sauce and mozzarella cheese, and bake until bubbly. Serve with mixed green salad or a serving of whole wheat pasta.

1.5 Mediterranean Chicken and Vegetable Skewers:

Thread chunks of chicken breast, cherry tomatoes, bell peppers, onions, and zucchini onto skewers. Brush with a mixture of olive oil, lemon juice, garlic, and oregano, then grill until chicken is cooked through and vegetables are tender. Serve with couscous or quinoa tabbouleh.

2. One-Pan Meals for Easy Cleanup:

2.1 Sheet Pan Honey Mustard Chicken and Vegetables:

Toss chicken breast, baby potatoes, Brussels sprouts, and carrots with a honey mustard marinade. Spread on a sheet pan and roast until chicken is cooked through and vegetables are tender.

2.2 One-Pot Quinoa Primavera:

Cook quinoa in vegetable broth with diced onions, bell peppers, zucchini, and cherry tomatoes until tender. Stir in fresh herbs like basil and parsley, and top with grated Parmesan cheese before serving.

2.3 Skillet Shrimp and Vegetable Fajitas:

Saute shrimp with bell peppers, onions, and fajita seasoning in a large skillet until shrimp are cooked through and vegetables are tender-crisp. Serve with warm whole wheat tortillas and your favorite toppings like salsa, guacamole, and Greek yogurt.

2.4 One-Pan Teriyaki Tofu and Broccoli:

Bake tofu cubes and broccoli florets tossed in a homemade teriyaki sauce on a sheet pan until tofu is crispy and broccoli is tender. Serve over brown rice and garnish with sesame seeds and green onions.

2.5 Sausage and Potato Bake:

Toss sliced sausage, baby potatoes, bell peppers, and onions with olive oil and Italian seasoning on a sheet pan. Roast until sausage is browned and potatoes are tender. Serve with a side of steamed green beans or a mixed green salad.

3. Vegetarian and Vegan Dinner Options:

3.1 Vegetable Curry with Chickpeas:

Simmer chickpeas, cauliflower, bell peppers, onions, and spinach in a flavorful coconut milk-based curry sauce. Season with curry powder, turmeric, and ginger, and serve over brown rice or quinoa.

3.2 Lentil and Sweet Potato Shepherd's Pie:

Cook lentils with diced sweet potatoes, carrots, onions, and garlic in vegetable broth until tender. Top with mashed sweet potatoes and bake until bubbly and golden brown.

3.3 Mushroom and Spinach Stuffed Portobello Mushrooms:

Remove stems from portobello mushrooms and fill with a mixture of sauteed mushrooms, spinach, garlic, and breadcrumbs. Bake until mushrooms are tender and filling is heated through.

3.4 Vegan Chickpea and Vegetable Stir-Fry:

Stir-fry chickpeas with a variety of colorful vegetables such as broccoli, bell peppers, snap peas, and carrots in a sesame-ginger sauce. Serve over quinoa or brown rice for a nutritious and satisfying meal.

3.5 Butternut Squash and Black Bean Enchiladas:

Fill corn tortillas with a mixture of roasted butternut squash, black beans, diced onions, and spices. Roll up and place in a baking dish, then top with enchilada sauce and bake until bubbly. Serve with a side of Mexican-style rice and guacamole.

3.6 Vegan Lentil and Vegetable Soup:

Simmer lentils with diced tomatoes, carrots, celery, onions, and garlic in vegetable broth until tender. Add chopped kale or spinach and season with herbs like thyme and rosemary. Serve with a slice of whole grain bread or a side salad for a complete meal.

3.7 Vegetable Stir-Fry with Tofu and Cashews:

Stir-fry cubes of tofu with a variety of colorful vegetables such as bell peppers, broccoli, snap peas, and carrots in a flavorful sauce made with soy sauce, ginger, garlic, and sesame oil. Toss in cashews for added crunch and protein. Serve over brown rice or quinoa.

3.8 Vegan Mediterranean Stuffed Peppers:

Halve bell peppers and remove seeds, then fill with a mixture of cooked quinoa, diced tomatoes, olives, artichoke hearts, and chopped fresh herbs like parsley and basil. Bake until peppers are tender and filling is heated through.

3.9 Chickpea and Vegetable Curry with Coconut Milk:

Simmer chickpeas with diced potatoes, carrots, bell peppers, onions, and cauliflower in a creamy coconut milk-based curry sauce. Season with curry powder, turmeric, and cumin for a warm and comforting meal. Serve over basmati rice or with naan bread.

3.10 Vegan Lentil Sloppy Joes:

Cook lentils with diced onions, bell peppers, and garlic in a tangy tomato-based sauce flavored with spices like chili powder, paprika, and cumin. Serve on whole grain buns or lettuce wraps and top with sliced avocado or pickles for added flavor.

These vegetarian and vegan dinner options are not only delicious but also packed with nutrients and flavor. They are perfect for anyone looking to incorporate more plant-based meals into their diet or for those following a vegetarian or vegan lifestyle. Enjoy experimenting with these recipes and making them your own!

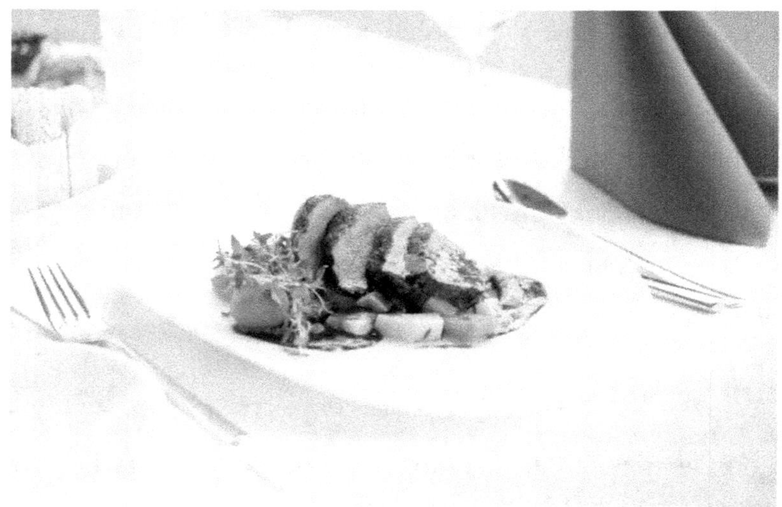

CHAPTER SIX

Snacks and Appetizers

1. Healthy Snacks to Keep Blood Sugar Stable

Keeping blood sugar stable is essential for maintaining energy levels and overall health. These are healthy snacks that can help stabilize blood sugar levels:

1.1 Apple slices with almond butter: The combination of fiber from the apple and healthy fats and protein from almond butter helps maintain steady blood sugar levels.

1.2 Greek yogurt with berries: Greek yogurt is high in protein and low in sugar, while berries provide fiber and antioxidants.

1.3 Hummus and veggie sticks: Hummus is a good source of protein and healthy fats, and pairing it with colorful vegetables adds fiber and nutrients.

1.4 Hard-boiled eggs: Eggs are rich in protein and healthy fats, which can help stabilize blood sugar levels.

1.5 Cottage cheese with cucumber slices: Cottage cheese is a low-carb, high-protein snack, and adding cucumber slices provides extra hydration and crunch.

1.6 Mixed nuts: Nuts like almonds, walnuts, and pistachios are packed with healthy fats, protein, and fiber, making them an excellent snack for stabilizing blood sugar.

1.7 Edamame: Edamame is a great source of plant-based protein and fiber, which can help keep blood sugar levels steady.

1.8 Cherry tomatoes with mozzarella cheese: This snack combines the protein and calcium from mozzarella cheese with the vitamins and antioxidants from cherry tomatoes.

1.9 Avocado toast on whole grain bread: Avocado is rich in healthy fats and fiber, and pairing it with whole grain bread adds additional fiber and nutrients.

1.10 Tuna lettuce wraps: Tuna is a lean source of protein, and wrapping it in lettuce leaves instead of bread helps keep the snack low in carbohydrates.

1.11 Chia seed pudding: Chia seeds are high in fiber and omega-3 fatty acids, which can help stabilize blood sugar levels when soaked in liquid to form a pudding.

1.12 Turkey and cheese roll-ups: Roll slices of turkey breast with cheese for a protein-rich snack that's low in carbohydrates.

1.13 Steamed edamame sprinkled with sea salt: This simple snack is high in protein and fiber, making it a great option for stabilizing blood sugar levels.

1.14 Roasted chickpeas: Chickpeas are a good source of protein and fiber, and roasting them with spices creates a crunchy, satisfying snack.

1.15 Veggie omelette muffins: Make mini omelettes in a muffin tin using eggs and chopped vegetables like bell peppers, spinach, and mushrooms for a protein-packed snack that's also full of vitamins and minerals

2. Appetizers for Entertaining or Quick Bites:

2.1 Caprese skewers: Cherry tomatoes, mozzarella balls, and fresh basil leaves skewered and drizzled with balsamic glaze.

2.2 Mini spinach and feta quiches: Bite-sized quiches made with spinach, feta cheese, and eggs baked in muffin tins.

2.3 Bruschetta: Bruschetta is a dish made of toasted baguette pieces with chopped tomatoes, garlic, basil, and olive oil on top.

2.4 Stuffed mushrooms: Mushroom caps filled with a mixture of cream cheese, garlic, herbs, and breadcrumbs, then baked until golden brown.

2.5 Smoked salmon cucumber bites: Thinly sliced cucumber rounds topped with smoked salmon, cream cheese, and fresh dill.

2.6 Mini meatballs: Bite-sized meatballs made with ground beef or turkey, breadcrumbs, herbs, and spices, served with a dipping sauce.

2.7 Vegetable spring rolls: Rice paper rolls filled with a variety of fresh vegetables like carrots, cucumbers, lettuce, and herbs, served with a peanut or hoisin dipping sauce.

2.8 Spicy shrimp cocktail: Chilled shrimp served with a spicy cocktail sauce made with horseradish, ketchup, Worcestershire sauce, and lemon juice.

2.9 Mini chicken skewers: Marinated chicken pieces threaded onto skewers and grilled until cooked through, served with a dipping sauce.

1.10 Guacamole deviled eggs: Hard-boiled eggs filled with a mixture of mashed avocado, lime juice, cilantro, and spices, topped with a sprinkle of paprika.

3. Portable Snacks for On-the-Go:

3.1 Trail mix: A mixture of nuts, seeds, and dried fruit for a convenient and satisfying snack.

3.2 Whole fruit: Apples, bananas, oranges, or any other fruit that's easy to eat on the go.

3. 3String cheese: Individual portions of string cheese for a quick source of protein and calcium.

3.4 Rice cakes with almond butter: Light and crunchy rice cakes spread with almond butter for a satisfying snack.

3.4 Veggie sticks with hummus: Carrot, celery, and cucumber sticks paired with hummus for a nutritious and portable snack.

3.5 Hard-boiled eggs: Pre-cooked and easy to transport, hard-boiled eggs are a great source of protein.

3.6 Greek yogurt cups: Single-serving containers of Greek yogurt for a protein-rich snack that's easy to eat on the go.

3.7 Seaweed snacks: Crispy sheets of roasted seaweed seasoned with salt or other flavors for a savory and portable snack.

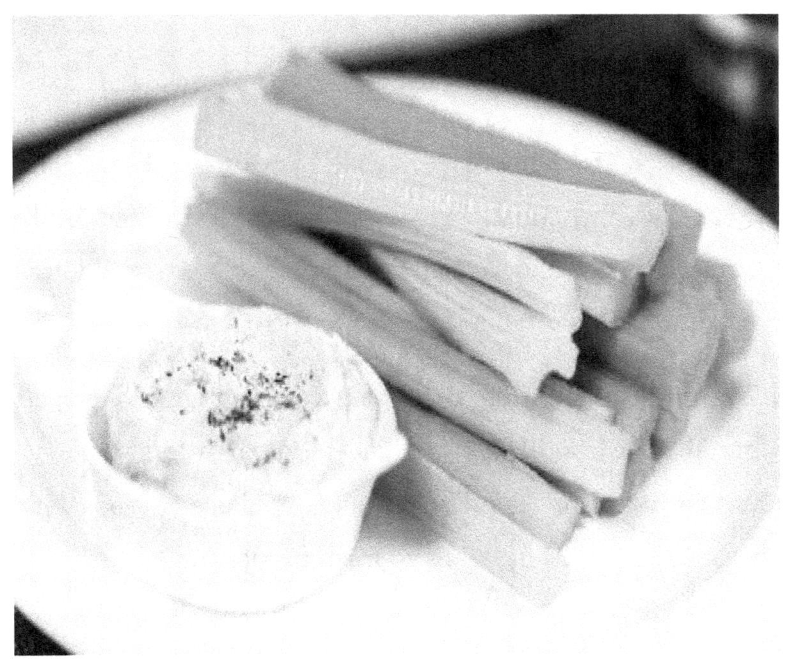

Hummus and veggie sticks

CHAPTER SEVEN

Desserts and Treats

1. Sugar-Free Desserts for Sweet Cravings:

1.1 Sugar-Free Chocolate Avocado Mousse: Blend ripe avocados with cocoa powder, a splash of almond milk, vanilla extract, and a natural sweetener like stevia or erythritol until smooth and creamy.

1.2 Chia Seed Pudding: Mix chia seeds with unsweetened almond milk, vanilla extract, and a sugar-free sweetener, then let it sit in the fridge until thickened. Top with unsweetened coconut flakes or fresh berries.

1.3 Sugar-Free Peanut Butter Cookies: Combine natural peanut butter, almond flour, a sugar substitute like monk fruit sweetener, and an egg. Roll into balls, flatten with a fork, and bake until golden brown.

1.4 Coconut Flour Banana Bread: Use coconut flour, ripe bananas, eggs, vanilla extract, and a sugar substitute to make a moist and delicious banana bread that's free from refined sugars.

1.5 Sugar-Free Greek Yogurt Parfait: Layer unsweetened Greek yogurt with fresh berries, nuts, and a drizzle of sugar-free syrup or a sprinkle of cinnamon for a satisfying dessert.

1.6 Sugar-Free Cheesecake Bites: Make a cheesecake filling using cream cheese, Greek yogurt, vanilla extract, and a sugar substitute. Spoon into mini muffin tins and chill until set.

1.7 No-Bake Almond Butter Energy Balls: Mix almond butter, rolled oats, chia seeds, unsweetened shredded coconut, vanilla extract, and a sugar-free sweetener. shape into balls and refrigerate until solid.

2.Fruit-Based Desserts and Frozen Treats:

2.1 Strawberry Banana Nice Cream: Blend frozen strawberries and bananas until smooth and creamy for a naturally sweet frozen treat.

2.2 Mango Coconut Popsicles: Blend ripe mango with coconut milk and a touch of lime juice, then pour into popsicle molds and freeze until solid.

2.3 Grilled Pineapple with Cinnamon: Grill pineapple slices until caramelized, then sprinkle with cinnamon for a simple and flavorful dessert.

2.4 Berry Frozen Yogurt Bark: Spread Greek yogurt onto a baking sheet, top with fresh berries, and freeze until firm. Break into pieces to enjoy as a cool snack.

2.5 Watermelon Lime Sorbet: Blend frozen watermelon chunks with lime juice and a bit of honey or agave syrup until smooth, then freeze until firm.

2.6 Peach Yogurt Popsicles: Puree ripe peaches with Greek yogurt and a splash of orange juice, then pour into popsicle molds and freeze until set.

2.7 Kiwi Lime Fruit Salad: Combine sliced kiwi with fresh lime juice and a drizzle of honey or agave syrup for a tangy and sweet fruit salad.

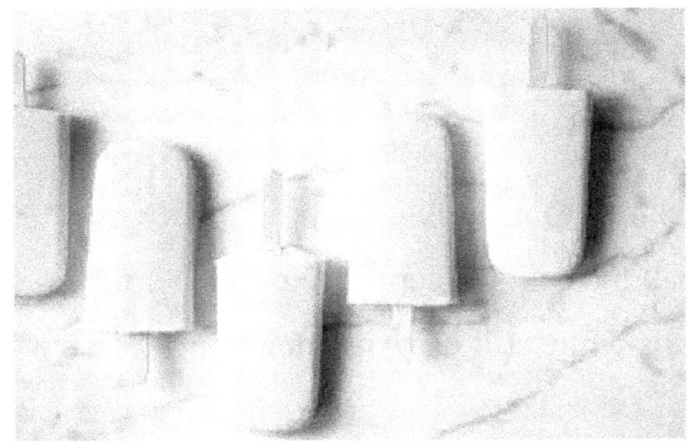

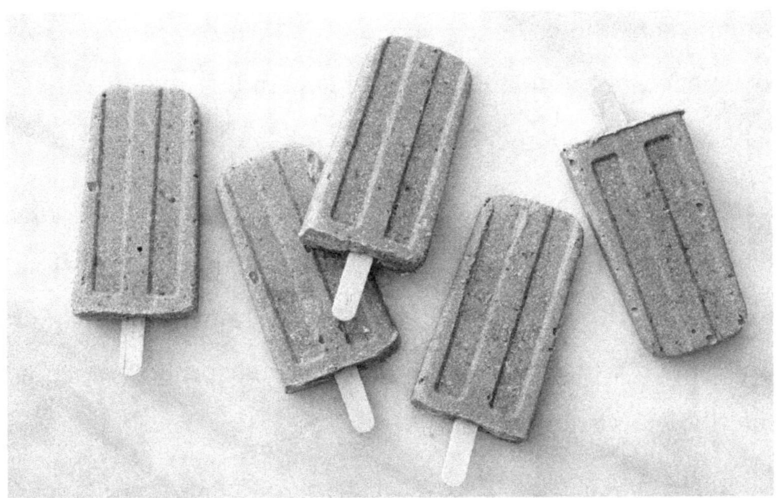

The Baking Tips for Making Diabetes-Friendly Treats

When it comes to making diabetes-friendly treats, there are several baking tips to keep in mind to help manage blood sugar levels while still enjoying delicious desserts. Here are some key tips:

Use sugar substitutes: Instead of traditional sugar, opt for sugar substitutes like stevia, erythritol, monk fruit sweetener, or xylitol. These sugar substitutes add sweetness without raising blood sugar levels.

Choose whole grain flours: Use whole grain flours like whole wheat flour, almond flour, coconut flour, or oat flour instead of refined white flour. Whole grain flour contains more fiber, which helps slow down the absorption of sugar into the bloodstream.

Add fiber-rich ingredients: Incorporate fiber-rich ingredients like fruits, vegetables, nuts, and seeds into your recipes. Fiber helps slow down the digestion of carbohydrates, leading to more stable blood sugar levels.

Reduce added fats: While fats can be beneficial in moderation, excessive fat intake can lead to weight gain and insulin resistance. Opt for healthier fats like olive oil, avocado, nuts, and seeds, and use them sparingly in your recipes.

Watch portion sizes: Pay attention to portion sizes when enjoying diabetes-friendly treats. Even though they may be lower in sugar and carbohydrates, consuming large portions can still affect blood sugar levels. To assist with blood sugar management, abide by the recommended serving sizes.

Experiment with alternative ingredients: Get creative with alternative ingredients to replace high-carb and high-sugar components in traditional recipes. For example, use mashed avocado or banana as a replacement for butter or oil in baked goods, or try using unsweetened applesauce to add moisture and sweetness.

Limit added toppings and fillings: Be mindful of added toppings and fillings that can contribute to excess sugar and calories. Instead of sugary frosting, consider using Greek yogurt or whipped coconut cream for a lighter topping. For fillings, opt for fresh fruits or sugar-free preserves.

Monitor blood sugar response: Everyone's body responds differently to different foods, so it's essential to monitor your blood sugar levels after consuming diabetes-friendly treats. Keep track of how certain ingredients and recipes affect your blood sugar and adjust accordingly.

By following these baking tips and making mindful ingredient choices, you can enjoy delicious diabetes-friendly treats while still maintaining stable blood sugar levels

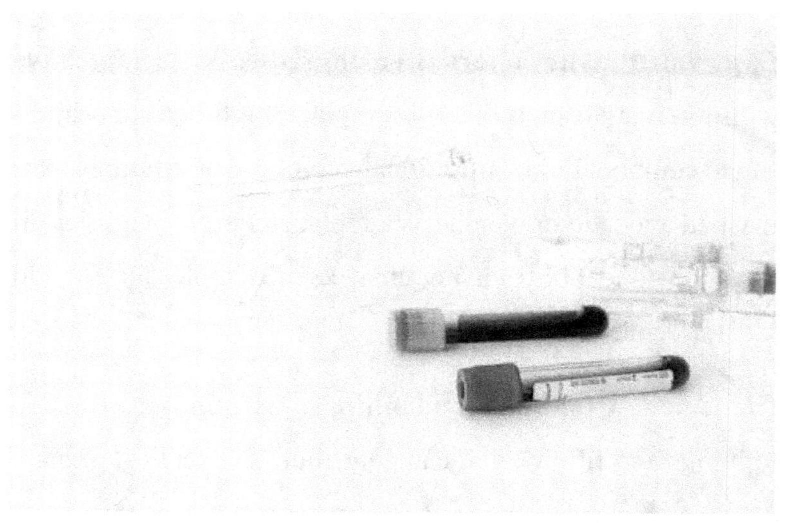

CHAPTER EIGHT

Hydrating Drinks Without Added Sugars:

Water: Plain water is the best choice for staying hydrated without any added sugars or calories.

Herbal teas: Herbal teas like chamomile, peppermint, or hibiscus are naturally caffeine-free and sugar-free options for hydration.

Sparkling water: Carbonated water with no added sugars or flavors can be a refreshing alternative to plain water.

Coconut water: Coconut water is naturally hydrating and contains electrolytes like potassium, making it a good choice for replenishing fluids.

Infused water: Add slices of fruits like lemon, lime, cucumber, or berries to water for a flavorful twist without added sugars.

Vegetable juice: Freshly squeezed vegetable juices, like cucumber or celery juice, can be hydrating and nutritious without added sugars.

Low-Carb Smoothies and Shakes:

Green smoothie: Blend spinach or kale with unsweetened almond milk, avocado, and a small amount of low-carb fruits like berries or green apple.

Berry protein shake: Blend unsweetened almond milk with a scoop of protein powder, mixed berries, and a handful of spinach for a low-carb, high-protein shake.

Avocado smoothie: Blend ripe avocado with unsweetened coconut milk, vanilla extract, and a sugar substitute like stevia or erythritol for a creamy and low-carb smoothie.

Peanut butter banana shake: Blend unsweetened almond milk with natural peanut butter, a small amount of banana, and a scoop of protein powder for a satisfying and low-carb shake.

Chocolate almond butter smoothie: Blend unsweetened almond milk with cocoa powder, almond butter, and a sugar substitute for a decadent and low-carb treat.

Coconut berry smoothie: Blend coconut milk with mixed berries, unsweetened shredded coconut, and a scoop of protein powder for a tropical-flavored, low-carb smoothie.

Coffee, Tea, and Other Diabetes-Friendly Beverages:

Black coffee: Plain black coffee is a zero-calorie, zero-carb beverage that can be enjoyed hot or cold.

Unsweetened tea: Whether black, green, or herbal, unsweetened tea is a great option for diabetes-friendly hydration.

Sparkling water with a splash of citrus: Add a squeeze of lemon, lime, or orange to sparkling water for a refreshing and sugar-free beverage.

Iced herbal tea: Brew herbal tea like chamomile or peppermint and chill it for a refreshing and caffeine-free option.

Matcha latte with unsweetened almond milk: Whisk matcha powder with unsweetened almond milk and a sugar substitute for a diabetes-friendly alternative to traditional lattes.

Turmeric latte with coconut milk: Heat coconut milk with turmeric, cinnamon, and a pinch of black pepper for a warming and anti-inflammatory beverage.

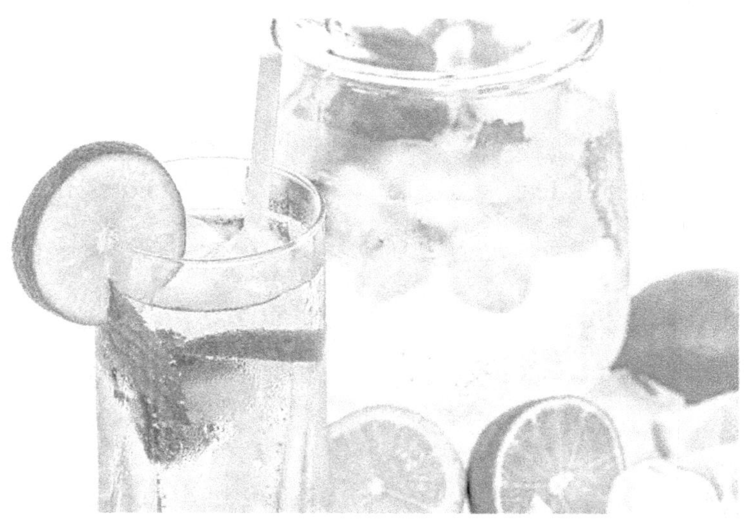

CHAPTER NINE

Meal Planning and Tips

Meal planning is a crucial aspect of managing diabetes as it helps regulate blood sugar levels and promotes overall health. Here's a detailed explanation of meal planning and tips for diabetics:

Understand Carbohydrate Counting: Carbohydrates have the most significant impact on blood sugar levels. For diabetics, it's essential to monitor carbohydrate intake and distribute it evenly throughout the day. Carbohydrate counting involves keeping track of the grams of carbohydrates consumed per meal and snack. This helps individuals manage their blood sugar levels more effectively.

Focus on Whole Foods: Emphasize whole, nutrient-dense foods in your diet, such as fruits, vegetables, lean proteins, whole grains, and healthy fats. These foods provide essential nutrients, fiber, and antioxidants, which support overall health and help stabilize blood sugar levels.

Portion Control: Controlling portion sizes is crucial for managing blood sugar levels and weight. Use measuring cups, spoons, or visual cues to portion out food accurately. Eating smaller, balanced meals and snacks throughout the day can help prevent spikes in blood sugar levels.

Foods with a low GI take longer to break down and absorb, which gradually raises blood sugar levels. Foods with a low GI take longer to break down and absorb, which gradually raises blood sugar levels. Include more low-GI foods such as non-starchy vegetables, legumes, whole grains, and nuts in your meals.

Balanced Meals: Try to eat meals that are well-balanced, with a mix of healthy fats, proteins, and carbs. Protein and fat help slow down the absorption of carbohydrates, preventing rapid spikes in blood sugar levels. For example, pair carbohydrates like whole grains or fruits with lean proteins such as chicken, fish, tofu, or beans, and incorporate healthy fats like olive oil, avocado, or nuts.

Limit Added Sugars and Processed Foods: Minimize the consumption of foods and beverages high in added sugars, refined carbohydrates, and processed ingredients. These can cause rapid fluctuations in blood sugar levels and contribute to weight gain and other health issues. whenever possible choose for whole, minimally processed foods

Stay Hydrated: Drinking plenty of water throughout the day is essential for overall health and helps regulate blood sugar levels. Aim for at least 8 glasses of water per day, and choose water over sugary beverages like soda, juice, or sweetened teas.

Be Mindful of Alcohol: Moderate alcohol consumption can be included in a diabetic meal plan, but it's essential to be mindful of its effects on blood sugar levels. Consuming alcohol in a large quantity or an empty stomach can lower blood sugar levels. Limit alcohol intake and consume it with food to minimize its impact on blood sugar levels.

Two Weekly Meal Plans for Diabetes Management

A 14-day meal plan for diabetes management requires careful consideration of nutritional needs, portion sizes, and balanced meals. Here's a sample meal plan that incorporates a variety of foods and flavors while focusing on managing blood sugar levels.

Week 1

Day 1:

Breakfast: Greek yogurt with berries and a sprinkle of chopped nuts

Snack: Carrot sticks with hummus

Lunch: Mixed greens, cucumber, balsamic vinaigrette, and cherry tomatoes with Grilled Chicken salad

Snack: Apple slices with almond butter

Dinner: Cooked salmon with steamed broccoli and quinoa

Day 2:

Breakfast: Spinach and feta omelette with whole-grain toast

Snack: Celery sticks with peanut butter

Lunch: Mix lettuce, tomato, mustard, and pieces of turkey with avocado, and wrap in whole wheat tortilla,

Snack: Greek yogurt with sliced almonds

Dinner: Stir-fried tofu with bell peppers, snap peas, and brown rice

Day 3:

Breakfast: Overnight oats made with rolled oats, unsweetened almond milk, chia seeds, and sliced strawberries

Snack: Handful of mixed nuts

Lunch: Quinoa salad with chickpeas, diced bell peppers, cucumber, feta cheese, and lemon vinaigrette

Snack: Cottage cheese with pineapple chunks

Dinner: Roasted asparagus with Grilled shrimp skewers and sweet potato wedges

Day 4:

Breakfast: Mashed avocado and poached eggs with Whole grain toast

Snack: Cherry tomatoes with mozzarella cheese

Lunch: A side of mixed greens salad with Lentil soup.

Snack: Banana with a small handful of walnuts

Dinner: Cooked chicken breast with roasted Brussels sprouts and wild rice

Day 5:

Breakfast: Smoothie made with spinach, banana, unsweetened almond milk, and protein powder

Snack: Edamame pods

Lunch: Tuna salad stuffed in half an avocado, served with cucumber slices

Snack: Hard-boiled egg

Dinner: Beef stir-fry with broccoli, bell peppers, and snap peas, served over cauliflower rice

Day 6:

Breakfast: Cottage cheese with diced peaches and a sprinkle of cinnamon

Snack: Celery sticks with cream cheese

Lunch: Veggie wrap with hummus, shredded carrots, cucumber, spinach, and whole wheat tortilla

Snack: Greek yogurt with a drop of honey

Dinner: Baked cod with roasted zucchini and quinoa pilaf

Day 7:

Breakfast: Scrambled eggs with spinach and tomatoes, served with a slice of whole-grain toast

Snack: Handful of almonds

Lunch: Chicken Caesar salad with romaine lettuce, grilled chicken breast, cherry tomatoes, Parmesan cheese, and Caesar dressing (use a light dressing or make your own)

Snack: Apple slices with peanut butter

Dinner: Turkey meatballs with marinara sauce, served over spaghetti squash

This meal plan provides a variety of nutrient-dense foods while focusing on balanced meals and snacks to help manage blood sugar levels. Adjust portion sizes and food choices as needed based on individual dietary preferences, nutritional needs, and blood sugar monitoring. It's also essential to stay hydrated throughout the day by drinking plenty of water and other sugar-free beverages.

Week 2.

Breakfast: Mix spinach and tomatoes with Scrambled eggs and serve with whole-grain toast

Snack: Greek yogurt with mixed berries

Lunch: Turkey and avocado wrap with lettuce and whole wheat tortilla

Snack: Carrot sticks with hummus

Dinner: roasted asparagus and quinoa with Baked salmon.

Day 2:

Breakfast: Overnight oats with almond milk, chia seeds, and sliced strawberries

Snack: Handful of almonds

Lunch: Add cucumber, tomato, feta cheese, lemon vinaigrette, and Quinoa salad with chickpeas,

Snack: Apple slices with peanut butter

Dinner: Grilled chicken breast with steamed broccoli and brown rice

Day 3:

Breakfast: Greek yogurt parfait with granola and mixed berries

Snack: Celery sticks with cream cheese

Lunch: Lentil soup with a side of mixed greens salad

Snack: Cottage cheese with pineapple chunks

Dinner: Stir-fried tofu with bell peppers, snap peas, and cauliflower rice

Day 4:

Breakfast: Poached eggs and mashed avocado with Whole grain toast.

Snack: Cherry tomatoes with mozzarella cheese

Lunch: Turkey and vegetable stir-fry with brown rice

Snack: Hard-boiled egg

Dinner: Cooked cod with roasted Brussels sprouts and quinoa pilaf

Day 5:

Breakfast: Spinach and feta omelette with whole-grain toast

Snack: Edamame pods

Lunch: Chicken Caesar salad with romaine lettuce, grilled chicken breast, Parmesan cheese, and Caesar dressing

Snack: Handful of mixed nuts

Dinner: Beef stir-fry with broccoli, bell peppers, and snap peas, served over cauliflower rice

Day 6:

Breakfast: Smoothie made with spinach, banana, unsweetened almond milk, and protein powder

Snack: Sliced cucumber with hummus

Lunch: Veggie wrap with hummus, shredded carrots, cucumber, spinach, and whole wheat tortilla

Snack: Greek yogurt with a drop of honey

Dinner: Turkey meatballs with marinara sauce, served over spaghetti squash

Day 7:

Breakfast: Cottage cheese with diced peaches and a sprinkle of cinnamon

Snack: Almond butter on whole grain crackers

Lunch: Tuna salad stuffed in half an avocado, served with mixed greens

Snack: Fresh berries with whipped cream

Dinner: Grilled shrimp skewers with roasted vegetables and quinoa

.

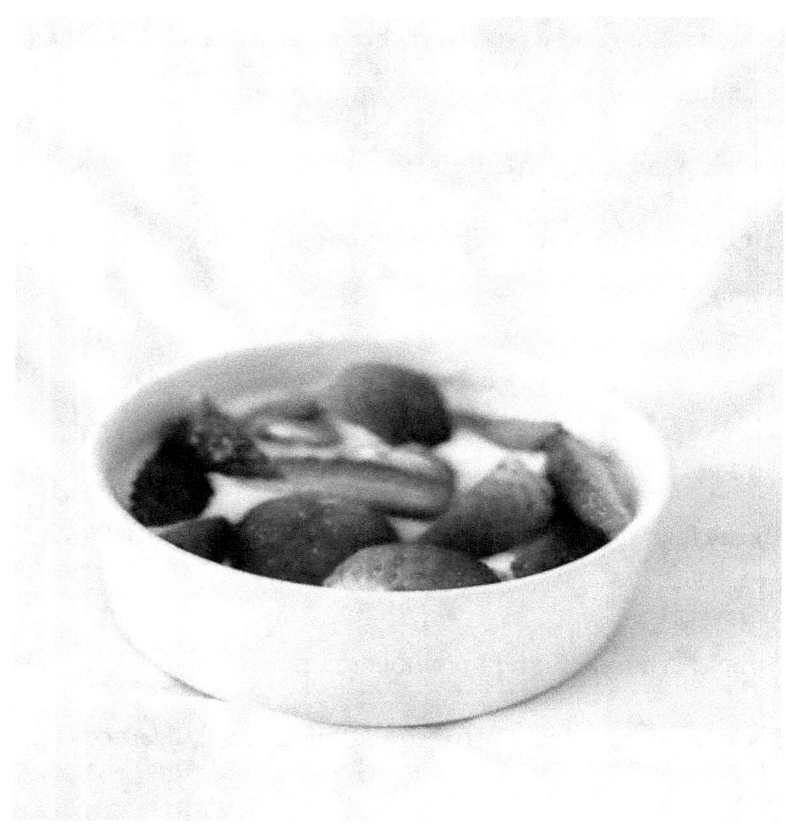

Regular Physical Activity: Incorporating regular physical activity into your routine can improve insulin sensitivity, lower blood sugar levels, and promote overall health. Aim for two times a week at least in strength training and at least 150 minutes of moderate-intensity aerobic activity per week.

Monitor Blood Sugar Levels: Regularly monitor your blood sugar levels as recommended by your healthcare provider. Keep track of how different foods, meals, and lifestyle factors affect your blood sugar levels and adjust your meal plan accordingly.

By following these meal planning tips and making healthy lifestyle choices, individuals with diabetes can better manage their condition and improve their overall quality of life. It's essential to work closely with a healthcare provider or registered dietitian to develop a personalized meal plan that meets individual nutritional needs and health goals

CHAPTER TEN

Sample grocery list

A sample grocery list tailored for managing diabetes. This list includes a variety of nutrient-dense foods to support blood sugar control and overall health:

Proteins:

Skinless chicken breast

Lean ground turkey or chicken

Salmon or other fatty fish

Tofu or tempeh

Eggs

Greek yogurt (unsweetened)

Cottage cheese (low-fat)

Beans (black beans, chickpeas, lentils)

Nuts and seeds (almonds, walnuts, chia seeds, flaxseeds)

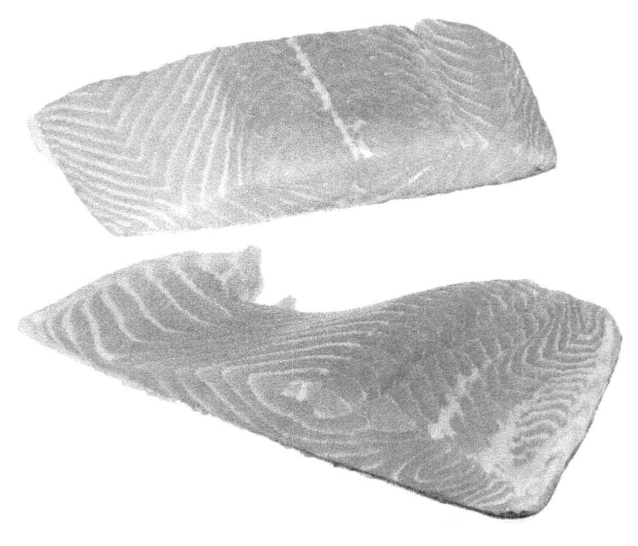

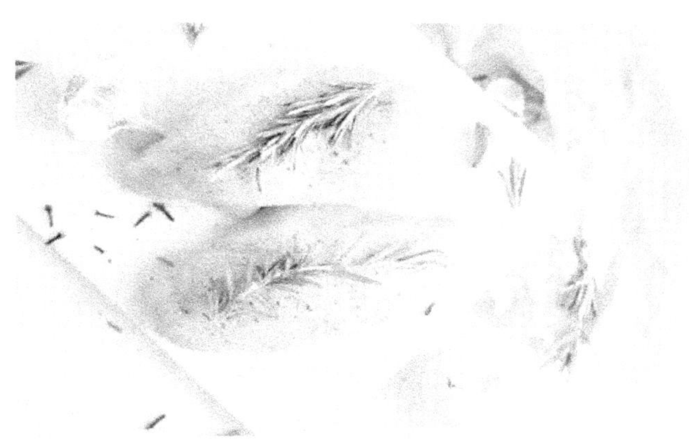

Leafy greens (spinach, kale, lettuce)

Cruciferous vegetables (broccoli, cauliflower, Brussels sprouts)

Bell peppers (red, green, yellow)

Tomatoes

Cucumbers

Carrots

Zucchini

Onions

Garlic

Avocado

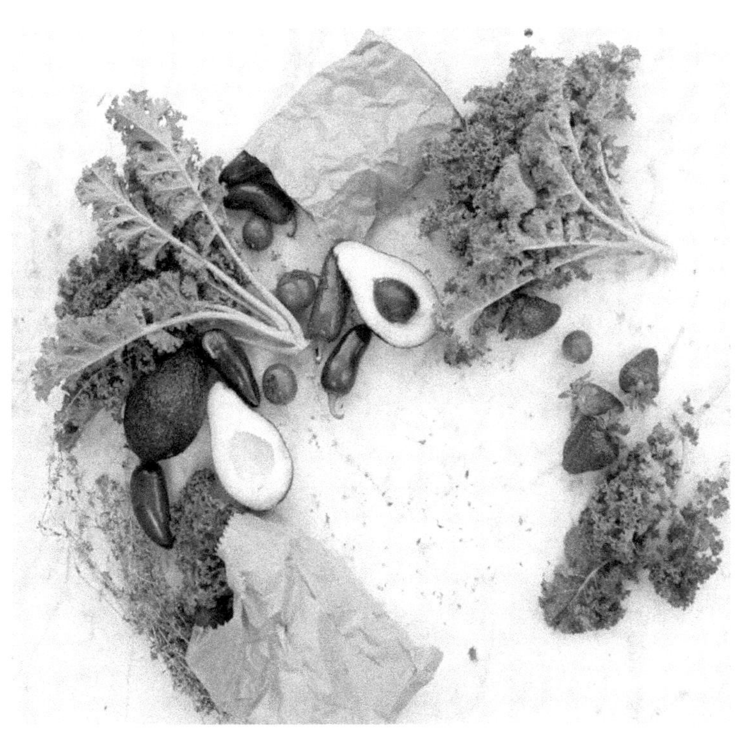

Fruits:

Berries (strawberries, blueberries, raspberries)

Apples

Oranges

Bananas

Peaches

Pears

Grapes

Kiwi

Lemons

Limes

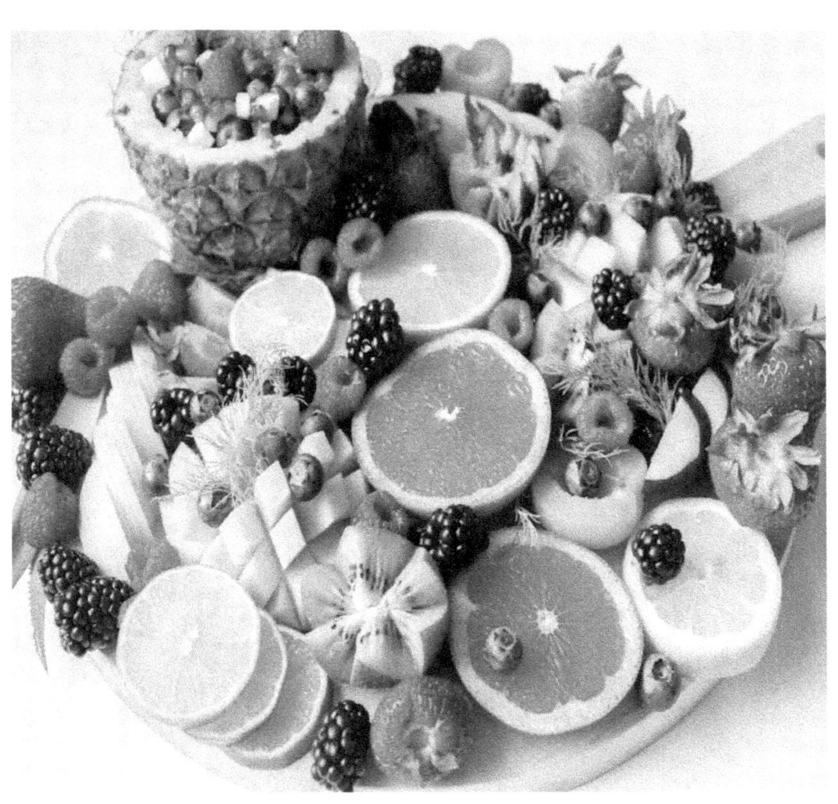

Whole Grains:

Quinoa

Brown rice

Whole wheat bread or wraps

Whole grain pasta

Oats

Barley

Farro

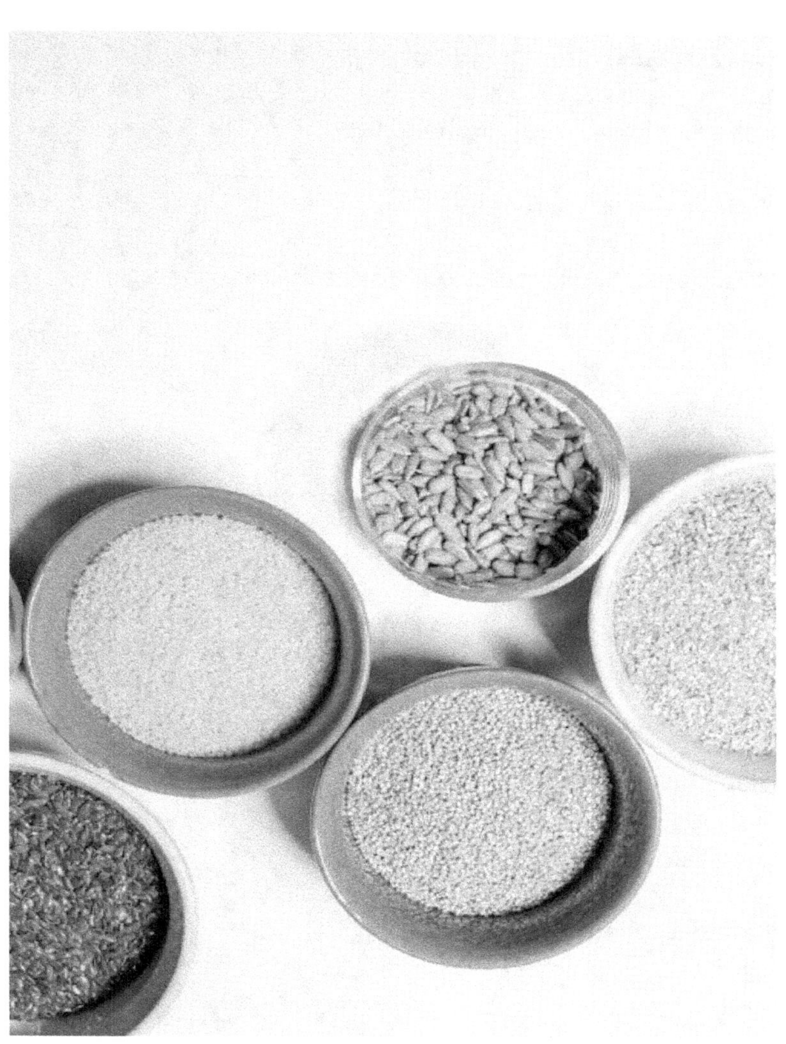

Dairy/Dairy Alternatives:

Unsweetened almond milk or soy milk

Low-fat cheese (mozzarella, feta)

Ricotta cheese (part-skim)

Butter or spreads made from olive oil or avocado

Beans and Legumes

Samples of legumes to pick up in canned, frozen, or dried form:

White beans

Lentils

Black beans

Garbanzo beans

Kidney beans

Pinto beans

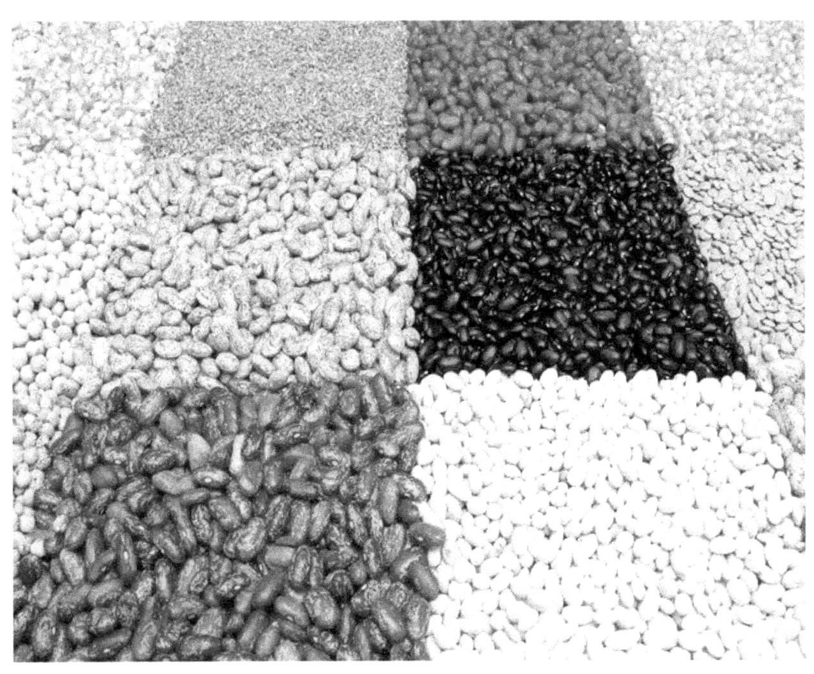

Healthy Fats:

Olive oil

Avocado oil

Coconut oil

Avocados

Nuts (almonds, walnuts, pecans)

Seeds (chia seeds, flaxseeds, pumpkin seeds)

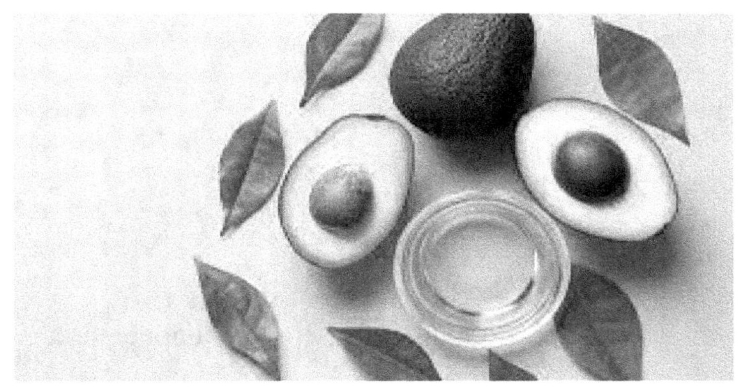

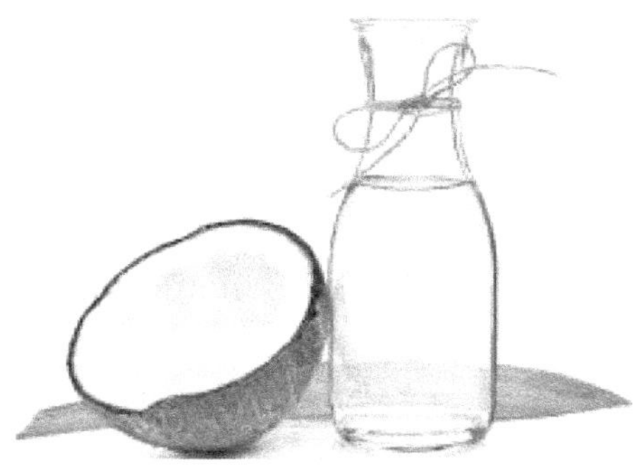

Other:

Hummus (plain)

Canned tuna or salmon (in water)

Low-sodium broth or stock

Herbs and spices (oregano, basil, cinnamon, turmeric, cumin)

Vinegar (balsamic vinegar, apple cider vinegar)

Unsweetened nut butter (almond butter, peanut butter)

It's essential to check food labels for added sugars and choose products with minimal processing. Additionally, be mindful of portion sizes and aim for a balanced diet that includes a variety of foods from each food group. Adjust quantities based on personal preferences and dietary needs.

Food to Avoid

Packaged and fast foods such as

Baked goods,

Sweets,

 Desserts

 Chips

White bread

White rice

White pasta and

Fried foods such as

French fries

sugary cereals

red meat

sugary drinks

processed meats

CHAPTER ELEVEN

Strategies for Eating Out with Diabetes

Eating out with diabetes can present challenges, but with careful planning and awareness, it's entirely manageable. Here are some strategies to help navigate restaurant dining while managing diabetes:

Research the Menu in Advance: Many restaurants now post their menus online. Before going out to eat, take some time to review the menu and identify healthier options that align with your dietary needs. Look for dishes that are grilled, baked, or steamed rather than fried, and choose items with lean proteins, vegetables, and whole grains.

Choose Restaurants Wisely: Opt for restaurants that offer a variety of healthier options and are willing to accommodate special dietary requests. Some restaurants may even have a separate section on their menu for healthier or lighter fare.

Be Mindful of Portions: Restaurant portion sizes are often larger than what you might eat at home. Consider sharing an entree with a dining companion or asking for a to-go box when your meal arrives and portioning out a smaller amount to eat.

Customize Your Order: Don't be afraid to ask for substitutions or modifications to meet your dietary needs. For example, request steamed vegetables instead of fries or a side salad instead of chips. Control the amount you use by asking that sauces and dressings should be put on the side.

Watch Out for Hidden Sugars and Carbs: Be mindful of hidden sugars and carbohydrates in sauces, dressings, and marinades. Opt for dishes with simple preparations and ask about the ingredients used in sauces and dressings.

Choose Water or Unsweetened Beverages: Skip sugary drinks like soda, sweet tea, or cocktails made with sugary mixers. Select water, unsweetened tea, or sparkling water with a lime or lemon splash as an alternative.

Limit Alcohol Consumption: If you choose to drink alcohol, do so in moderation and be aware of its effects on blood sugar levels. Stick to light beer, dry wine, or spirits mixed with sugar-free mixers, and avoid sugary cocktails and excessive consumption.

Practice Portion Control with Desserts: If you decide to indulge in dessert, consider sharing with others at the table or opting for a smaller portion. Look for lighter options like fresh fruit, sorbet, or a small piece of dark chocolate.

Monitor Blood Sugar Levels: Keep an eye on your blood sugar levels before, during, and after your meal, especially if you're trying new foods or dishes that may affect your blood sugar differently.

Don't Be Afraid to Speak Up: If you have specific dietary needs or concerns, don't hesitate to communicate them to your server or the restaurant staff. Most restaurants are willing to accommodate special requests to ensure a positive dining experience for all customers.

By following these strategies and making informed choices, you can enjoy dining out while still managing your diabetes effectively.

Tips for Success in Managing Diabetes Through Diet

Successfully managing diabetes through diet requires a combination of knowledge, planning, and consistent habits. There are some tips to help you succeed:

Educate Yourself: Learn about the basics of diabetes, including how different foods affect blood sugar levels, the importance of portion control, and how to read food labels. Understanding the fundamentals of nutrition empowers you to make informed choices about your diet.

Focus on Whole Foods: Base your diet around whole, minimally processed foods like fruits, vegetables, lean proteins, whole grains, and healthy fats. These foods are rich in nutrients, fiber, and antioxidants, which support overall health and help stabilize blood sugar levels.

Practice Portion Control: Pay attention to portion sizes and aim for balanced meals that include a combination of carbohydrates, protein, and healthy fats. Use measuring cups, spoons, or visual cues to portion out food accurately, and avoid oversized servings that can lead to spikes in blood sugar levels.

Choose Low-Glycemic Index Foods: Select foods with a low glycemic index (GI), which are digested and absorbed more slowly, resulting in gradual increases in blood sugar levels. Low-GI foods include non-starchy vegetables, legumes, whole grains, nuts, and seeds.

Balance Carbohydrates: Since carbohydrates have the most effect on blood sugar levels, it's critical to spread them out equally throughout the day. Choose complex carbohydrates like whole grains, fruits, and vegetables over refined carbohydrates, and pair them with lean proteins and healthy fats to help slow down digestion and minimize blood sugar spikes.

Be Mindful of Sugars and Sweeteners: Limit your intake of added sugars and opt for natural sweeteners like stevia, erythritol, or monk fruit when needed. Be cautious of foods labeled as "sugar-free" or "low-sugar," as they may still contain hidden sugars or high levels of artificial sweeteners.

Monitor Blood Sugar Levels: Regularly monitor your blood sugar levels as recommended by your healthcare provider to track how different foods, meals, and lifestyle factors affect your blood sugar. Keep a food diary to help identify patterns and make adjustments to your diet as needed.

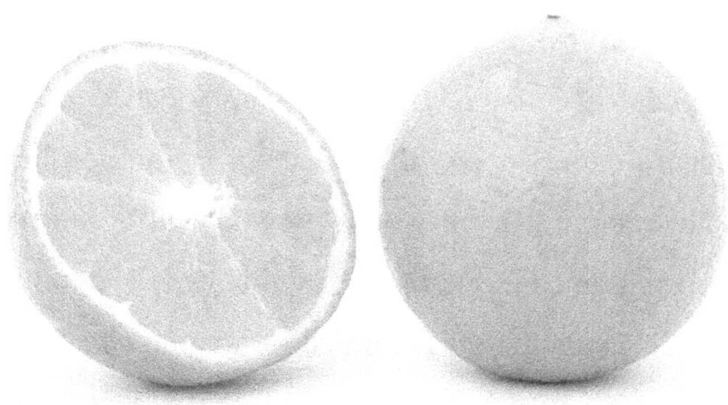

Conclusion:

Conclusively, the management of diabetes is a multifaceted journey that demands a holistic approach, unwavering commitment, and a profound understanding of the condition. Through this exploration, we've delved into various facets of diabetes management, from lifestyle adjustments to technological advancements, from psychological well-being to community support.

First and foremost, it's imperative to recognize that diabetes management is not a one-size-fits-all endeavor. Each individual's experience with diabetes is unique, influenced by factors ranging from genetic predispositions to socio-economic circumstances. Hence, a personalized approach is paramount, encompassing tailored treatment plans, dietary modifications, and exercise regimens that suit the specific needs of each person.

Throughout our discussion, the pivotal role of lifestyle modifications has emerged as a cornerstone of effective diabetes management. From adopting a balanced diet rich in whole foods to incorporating regular physical activity into daily routines, lifestyle changes wield tremendous power in controlling blood sugar levels and mitigating the risk of complications.

Moreover, initiatives promoting health education and awareness play a pivotal role in empowering individuals to make informed choices and take charge of their well-being. In tandem with lifestyle adjustments, technological innovations have revolutionized the landscape of diabetes management, offering an array of tools and resources to enhance monitoring, treatment, and support.

Continuous glucose monitoring (CGM) systems, insulin pumps, and mobile applications have empowered individuals with real-time insights and streamlined mechanisms for medication administration, fostering greater autonomy and flexibility in diabetes care.

However, amidst the wealth of technological advancements, it's essential not to overlook the intrinsic value of emotional and psychological well-being in diabetes management. The emotional toll of living with a chronic condition can be profound, encompassing feelings of anxiety, depression, and burnout. Thus, fostering a supportive environment that prioritizes mental health and encourages open communication is indispensable in promoting resilience and holistic wellness.

Furthermore, the significance of community support and peer networks cannot be overstated in the journey of diabetes management. Connecting with others who share similar experiences fosters a sense of camaraderie, dispels feelings of isolation, and provides invaluable opportunities for shared learning and encouragement.

Whether through support groups, online forums, or local meet-ups, the sense of solidarity derived from collective experiences is a potent catalyst for empowerment and growth. As we navigate the complex terrain of diabetes management, it's essential to recognize that challenges will inevitably arise, setbacks will occur, but perseverance and resilience will ultimately prevail.

By embracing a proactive mindset, leveraging the resources at our disposal, and cultivating a supportive ecosystem of care, we can navigate the intricacies of diabetes with grace and fortitude.

In closing, the management of diabetes is not merely about controlling blood sugar levels; it's about reclaiming agency over one's health, embracing a lifestyle of vitality, and cultivating a spirit of resilience in the face of adversity. Together, armed with knowledge, compassion, and unwavering determination, we can transcend the confines of diabetes and embark on a journey of vibrant health and well-being.

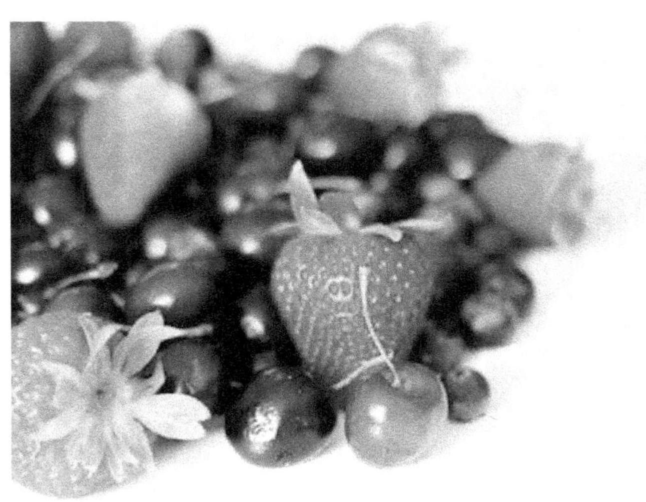

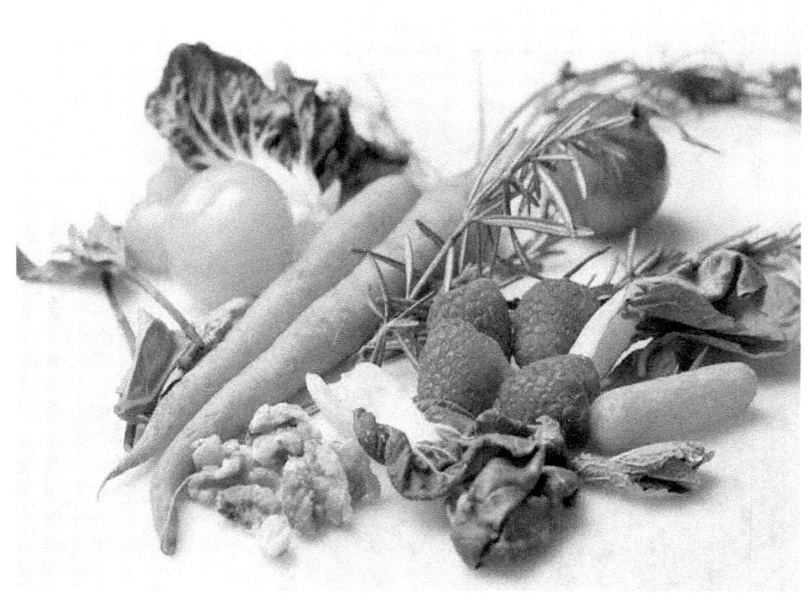